The Bad Egg

THE BAD EGG

Why Eggs Are Not a Health Food

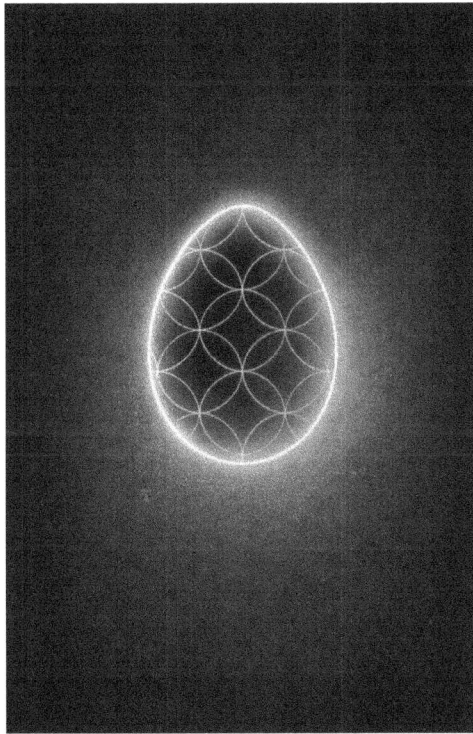

The Biological Evidence Linking
Egg Consumption To Chronic Illness

By Jesse J. Jacoby & Anthony Lowther

Soulspire Publishing
Truckee, CA, 96161

ISBN: 978-1-968660-36-9
Library of Congress Control Number: 2012921011
Dewey CIP: 641.563   **OCLC:** 213839254

Cover art, font, and layout are all original art by: Abdul Rehman

Wholesalers to book trade: Nelson's Books and Ingram
Available through Amazon.com, BarnesAndNoble.com

Dedication

This book is dedicated to those who chose to ask deeper questions about what they were taught to eat, and why. To the readers who sensed that something felt off long before the studies confirmed. To those who listened to their bodies when culture told them not to.

We dedicate these pages to every person who believes health should feel clear, light, and coherent, not congested, inflamed, or confusing.

We also dedicate this project to the future, where nourishment is guided by biology, integrity, and truth rather than tradition, marketing, or habit.

Acknowledgments

This book would not exist without the courage to question dietary norms that have long been protected by industry, nostalgia, and repetition. Writing about eggs as a biological stressor rather than a nutritional staple requires moving against deeply ingrained cultural beliefs, and that resistance is precisely why this work matters.

I extend deep gratitude to Anthony Lowther for his continued collaboration, research support, and willingness to examine nutrition through a biological and mechanistic lens rather than through ideology or convention. Our shared commitment to evidence, coherence, and metabolic truth has shaped this work at every level.

We acknowledge the physicians, researchers, and clinicians whose studies are cited throughout this book. Many of them did not set out to challenge dietary dogma, yet their data quietly does exactly that. Their work forms the backbone of this text.

Finally, thank you to the readers who have followed this series from *The Meat Effect* to *Dirty Dairy*, and now to *The Bad Egg*. This book exists because you were willing to look more closely, stay curious, and remain honest about what optimal health truly requires.

Framework of Findings

Introduction: Why Eggs Were Next

Eggs have occupied a unique and unusually protected position in modern nutrition. While red meat has increasingly been scrutinized for playing a significant role in cardiovascular disease and cancer, and dairy has been reevaluated for inflammatory and hormonal consequences, eggs have largely remained exempt from serious criticism. They are still widely described as clean, natural, and essential, particularly within health-conscious communities that otherwise avoid animal products.

This exemption did not arise because eggs are biologically benign. The omission from critique arose because eggs feel familiar. They are associated with simplicity, affordability, and tradition. They are woven into breakfast culture, athletic meal plans, and childhood memories. Over time, familiarity became compatibility.

Yet the human body does not evaluate food through nostalgia. Our system interprets food through digestion, microbial fermentation, metabolic processing, and immune response. When examined through these systems, eggs reveal a pattern of physiological stress that closely parallels, and at times exceeds, that of other animal-derived foods.

Eggs are reproductive material. Their biological purpose is to support the rapid growth of a developing organism. To serve that function, eggs contain concentrated proteins, dense fats, cholesterol, and signaling compounds designed to stimulate cellular proliferation. When introduced into the adult human digestive system, these compounds do not serve as nutrients in the conventional sense. They behave as metabolic burdens.

Unlike carbohydrates derived from fruits and vegetables, which are efficiently absorbed in the upper intestine, egg proteins are resistant to complete enzymatic breakdown. Significant portions reach the lower intestine intact, where they become substrate for proteolytic and acid-forming bacteria. These organisms metabolize egg proteins into secondary compounds such as ammonia, hydrogen sulfide, phenols, indoles, and biogenic amines. These byproducts compromise intestinal integrity, impair mitochondrial respiration in colon cells, and contribute to systemic inflammatory signaling once absorbed.

The problem does not disappear when eggs are consumed raw. While raw eggs avoid some of the toxic compounds created by cooking, they introduce a separate set of biological stressors. Raw egg whites contain avidin, a protein that binds biotin with extraordinary affinity, preventing absorption and increasing the risk of deficiency. Raw egg proteins are even more resistant to digestion than their cooked counterparts, increasing bacterial fermentation and toxin production in the colon. These effects occur regardless of bacterial contamination and are independent of food safety concerns.

Egg yolks further complicate digestion through their fat content. Dietary fat slows gastric emptying and delays protein digestion, increasing the likelihood that intact egg proteins reach the colon. High fat intake also enhances the absorption of bacterial endotoxins such as lipopolysaccharide into the bloodstream, a phenomenon known as metabolic endotoxemia. This low-grade inflammatory state has been strongly linked to insulin resistance, vascular dysfunction, and neuroinflammation.

Despite these mechanisms, eggs continue to be promoted as a nutritional necessity, often justified by claims of protein quality, choline content, or vitamin density. This book examines those claims in detail and evaluates them against current understanding of amino acid utilization, gut microbiome dynamics, lipid metabolism, and disease risk.

The decision to examine eggs as the third volume in this series was not ideological. After evaluating meat and dairy, eggs remained as the last major animal-derived food still widely perceived as harmless. Yet when the same biological framework is applied to digestion, fermentation, metabolism, inflammation, and long-term disease risk, the conclusions are consistent. Eggs are not required for human health, and their regular consumption imposes measurable physiological costs.

This book does not argue for purity, restriction, or dietary perfection. We push for coherence. Humans do not require reproductive material from another species to obtain protein, energy, or vitality. Amino acids are abundant in whole plant foods when consumed in adequate variety. Nutritional adequacy does not require metabolic compromise.

What follows is a biological examination of eggs as a dietary input. The analysis is grounded in physiology, biochemistry, and epidemiology rather than tradition or marketing. Each chapter builds upon the previous one, tracing the effects of egg consumption from digestion to cellular stress to chronic disease.

Eggs were next because they had to be. Not because they are uniquely harmful, but because they reveal how deeply dietary myths can persist when familiarity is mistaken for nourishment. Health improves by aligning with biology.

Part I: The Egg Illusion

Eggs occupy a unique psychological and cultural space in the modern diet. Unlike other animal-derived foods that have gradually been scrutinized for their health consequences, eggs continue to benefit from an assumption of innocence. They are framed as simple, natural, and nutritionally complete, often exempt from the concerns applied to meat, dairy, or processed foods.

This section examines how that exemption was constructed. Before eggs are evaluated biologically, they must be understood culturally. Dietary myths rarely persist because they are accurate. Most persist because they are repeated, normalized, and emotionally reinforced. Eggs are no exception.

The chapters that follow dismantle the illusion surrounding eggs by tracing how marketing, tradition, selective science, and repetition converged to position eggs as a health food. Only once this narrative is exposed can the biological evidence be examined clearly and without bias.

Lesson 1: The Cultural Halo Around Eggs

Marketing, Mythology, and the Breakfast Narrative

Eggs are one of the most heavily mythologized foods in the modern diet. Their reputation as a health staple is not the result of neutral scientific consensus, but of decades of strategic framing that positioned eggs as essential, wholesome, and biologically necessary. This framing has been so effective that eggs are often excluded from discussions about animal-derived foods altogether, despite sharing many of the same metabolic liabilities.

The cultural halo surrounding eggs is reinforced from an early age. Eggs are introduced as one of the first *"real"* foods, framed as gentle, nourishing, and strengthening. Breakfast culture has played a central role in normalizing daily egg consumption. The idea that a proper morning meal requires eggs has been repeated so frequently that the notion is rarely questioned. Over time, repetition has been mistaken for evidence.

Industry influence has played a decisive role in shaping this perception. Marketing campaigns funded by the egg industry have consistently emphasized protein quality, simplicity, and vitality while minimizing or omitting discussion of cholesterol, saturated fat, digestion, and disease risk. Phrases such as *"nature's perfect protein"* and *"nutritional powerhouse"* are not scientific conclusions. These are advertising constructs that have been absorbed into public consciousness as fact.

The athletic and fitness communities further amplified this narrative. Eggs became synonymous with strength, muscle development, and discipline. The visual symbolism of eggs as compact, self-contained units of nutrition made them appealing in performance-oriented spaces.

Rarely discussed in these settings were the downstream effects of repeated egg consumption on gut ecology, lipid metabolism, or inflammation. The focus remained fixed on macronutrient quantity rather than biological consequence.

Medical and nutritional institutions contributed to the halo by offering inconsistent and often contradictory guidance. For decades, dietary cholesterol was recognized as a contributor to cardiovascular disease. Later, emphasis shifted toward saturated fat, allowing eggs to regain favor by comparison. This reframing did not absolve eggs of their biological effects but redirected scrutiny elsewhere. Eggs benefited not from exoneration, but from distraction.

Cultural tradition further insulated eggs from critique. Foods associated with heritage and routine are often defended instinctively, even in the face of conflicting evidence. Eggs feel familiar, inexpensive, and comforting. These qualities create emotional resistance to reevaluation. When evidence challenges familiar foods, this is often perceived as an attack on identity rather than an invitation to examine biology.

This combination of marketing, institutional ambiguity, athletic endorsement, and cultural attachment created an environment in which eggs were rarely examined as a physiological input. Instead, they were treated as a default food, assumed to be safe until proven otherwise. This assumption reversed the burden of proof. Rather than asking whether eggs promote health, society assumed so and required overwhelming evidence to suggest otherwise.

The purpose of this book is not to vilify tradition, but to correct misplaced confidence. Foods do not earn their health status through repetition or nostalgia. They earn this through compatibility with human biology. Eggs have been shielded by perception far more than by physiology.

Lesson 2: How Eggs Became Food

Reproductive Biology Versus Human Nutrition

Eggs were not designed to nourish adult humans. They were designed to generate life. From a biological standpoint, this distinction is foundational, not philosophical. Eggs exist as reproductive vessels, engineered to support rapid cellular division, tissue formation, and embryonic growth. Their composition reflects that function precisely.

An egg contains concentrated proteins, dense lipids, cholesterol, and signaling molecules intended to stimulate proliferation. These compounds are beneficial to a developing embryo whose physiology is oriented toward accelerated growth. The adult human body, however, is not in a constant state of embryogenesis. We operate in a maintenance system, designed to preserve tissue integrity, regulate inflammation, and manage metabolic balance over decades. Foods that promote unchecked growth signaling are poorly matched to that task.

The historical adoption of eggs as food did not arise from biological necessity but from availability and convenience. In agricultural societies, eggs represented a readily accessible source of calories that required minimal processing. Their use expanded not because they were uniquely compatible with human physiology, but because they were abundant and easily collected. Over time, repeated use hardened into tradition, and tradition eventually became doctrine.

From a comparative biology perspective, humans are not ovivores. These are organisms who eat eggs as a significant part of their diet. Examples include snakes, lizards and monitor species, and some birds. No human digestive adaptation exists specifically for egg consumption.

The enzymes, gastric acidity, and intestinal transit times of the human digestive tract are optimized for fruits, roots, leaves, seeds, and other plant matter. Concentrated animal proteins and fats place a disproportionate burden on these systems, particularly when consumed frequently.

Egg proteins illustrate this mismatch clearly. They are structurally complex, resistant to complete digestion, and prone to reaching the colon intact. There, they become substrate for bacterial fermentation rather than nourishment for human cells. This is not a flaw in hygiene or preparation, but a reflection of biological incompatibility.

The argument that eggs are *"natural"* because they come from animals ignores a critical distinction. Natural does not mean appropriate. Venom is natural. Spoilage is natural. Reproductive tissue from another species may be natural, but that does not make this nutritionally coherent for humans. Biology evaluates compatibility, not origin.

The transition from scarcity-based diets to constant availability has further magnified this mismatch. Historically, egg consumption was sporadic. In modern diets, eggs are often eaten daily, sometimes multiple times per day. Reproductive material that once appeared occasionally is now treated as a staple. The human body experiences this not as nourishment, but as chronic exposure to growth-promoting compounds, dense fats, and digestion-resistant proteins.

Understanding eggs as reproductive material rather than food reframes the entire discussion. The question is no longer whether eggs contain nutrients. Most biological tissues contain nutrients. The question is whether those nutrients are delivered in a form and context that supports long-term human health. The evidence increasingly suggests they are not.

Lesson 3: The 'Perfect Protein' Myth

Bioavailability, Amino Acids, and Metabolic Reality

Eggs are frequently described as the *"perfect protein,"* a claim rooted in amino acid scoring systems rather than in lived human physiology. While egg protein contains a range of essential amino acids, the presence of amino acids alone does not determine nutritional value. What matters is digestion, absorption, utilization, and metabolic cost.

Protein bioavailability is often misunderstood. Scoring systems such as PDCAAS and DIAAS evaluate how closely a protein source matches human amino acid requirements under laboratory conditions. These models do not account for fermentation in the colon, endotoxin absorption, inflammatory signaling, or long-term disease risk. A protein can score highly on paper and perform poorly in the body.

Egg proteins are particularly problematic because of their resistance to digestion. Even when cooked, egg proteins frequently evade complete enzymatic breakdown. When raw, this resistance is even greater. Undigested protein entering the colon shifts the microbiome toward proteolytic species that generate toxic byproducts rather than beneficial short-chain fatty acids. This process undermines gut integrity and burdens detoxification pathways.

Plant-based amino acids behave differently. Fruits, vegetables, seeds, and greens deliver amino acids in lower concentrations but within a fiber-rich, antioxidant-dense matrix. This matrix supports gradual absorption in the small intestine, reduces fermentation toxicity, and promotes microbial diversity. The body assembles proteins from amino acids as needed and does not require pre-assembled animal protein to do so.

The fixation on protein quantity has obscured a more important truth, that excessive or poorly digested protein accelerates aging and disease. High protein intake stimulates insulin-like growth factor-1 (IGF-1), a hormone associated with increased cancer risk and reduced longevity when chronically elevated. Eggs, as a concentrated animal protein source, contribute disproportionately to this signaling pathway.

The myth of eggs as essential protein persists because nutrition is simplified into numbers rather than processes. Humans do not thrive on amino acid charts. They thrive on metabolic harmony. When protein intake exceeds digestive capacity or is delivered in a form that promotes fermentation and inflammation, theoretical completeness becomes irrelevant.

Eggs are not necessary to meet protein needs. Nor are they optimal. Adequate protein synthesis occurs readily in diets rich in whole plant foods, particularly when caloric sufficiency and variety are present. The body's requirement is for amino acids, not eggs.

When examined beyond marketing language and laboratory scoring, the *"perfect protein"* claim collapses. Eggs may look efficient on paper, but efficiency divorced from biological consequence is not health.

Part II: Digestion, Fermentation, & Gut Toxicity

Digestion is not merely a mechanical process of breaking food into smaller pieces. This is a biological negotiation between enzymes, microbes, immune tissue, and cellular metabolism. Foods that digest cleanly support energy production, microbial balance, and tissue repair. Foods that resist digestion become substrates for fermentation, inflammation, and toxicity.

Eggs fall into the latter category. Their proteins and fats challenge human digestive capacity in ways that are subtle in the short term but cumulative over time. This section traces what happens when eggs move through the gastrointestinal tract, how they alter microbial ecology, and why their digestion consistently produces inflammatory and toxic byproducts rather than nourishment.

Understanding these mechanisms is essential, because many of the long-term health effects associated with egg consumption originate in the gut, not the bloodstream.

Lesson 4: Egg Proteins & Digestive Resistance

Why Egg Proteins Are Poorly Broken Down

Egg proteins are structurally complex and unusually resistant to complete digestion. Unlike plant proteins, which are packaged with fiber, water, and protective phytochemicals, egg proteins arrive in a concentrated, isolated form. This concentration overwhelms digestive enzymes and increases the likelihood that intact or partially digested proteins will pass into the lower intestine.

The human digestive system relies on gastric acid and proteolytic enzymes such as pepsin and trypsin to break proteins into absorbable amino acids. Egg proteins, particularly ovalbumin and ovomucoid, resist these processes. Even under optimal digestive conditions, a significant fraction of egg protein remains incompletely digested. This resistance is amplified in individuals with reduced stomach acid, slowed motility, or compromised enzyme production, all of which are increasingly common.

Protein that escapes digestion in the small intestine becomes fuel for proteolytic bacteria in the colon. These bacteria metabolize amino acids not for human benefit, but for their own survival, producing metabolic byproducts that are biologically hostile to the host.

Repeated exposure to digestion-resistant proteins alters gut ecology over time. Microbial populations shift away from carbohydrate-fermenting species that produce beneficial short-chain fatty acids and toward protein-fermenting organisms that generate toxic metabolites. This shift compromises gut barrier integrity and increases inflammatory signaling.

Egg proteins are not uniquely problematic in isolation. They are problematic in context. Their concentration, resistance to digestion, and frequency of consumption combine to create a chronic burden on the digestive system. What appears to be a clean protein source on the plate becomes a source of microbial imbalance and toxicity once digestion fails.

Lesson 5: Raw Eggs – Uncooked Does Not Mean Safe

Avidin, Enzyme Inhibition, & Nutrient Interference

Raw eggs are often promoted as a cleaner or more natural alternative to cooked eggs. This assumption is based on the avoidance of heat-induced toxins rather than on an understanding of digestion. Raw eggs introduce distinct biological problems that persist regardless of food safety or bacterial contamination.

Raw egg whites contain avidin, a glycoprotein that binds biotin with extraordinary strength. Biotin is essential for fatty acid metabolism, glucose regulation, and nervous system function. When avidin binds biotin in the digestive tract, absorption is prevented entirely. This interaction occurs before nutrients reach circulation, rendering biotin intake from other foods ineffective in the presence of raw egg whites.

In addition to avidin, raw eggs contain enzyme inhibitors that interfere with trypsin and other digestive proteases. These inhibitors, which include ovomucoid, ovoinhibitor, ovostatin, and cystatin, further reduce protein digestion efficiency, increasing the volume of intact protein reaching the colon. Rather than nourishing human tissues, they fuel bacterial fermentation and toxin production.

Raw egg proteins are also more antigenic than cooked proteins. Their intact structure increases likelihood of immune recognition and inflammatory response, particularly in individuals with increased intestinal permeability. Over time, repeated immune activation contributes to low-grade inflammation and food sensitivity.

The appeal of raw eggs rests on a false dichotomy. Cooking eggs creates one set of problems and consuming them raw creates another.

Lesson 6: Acid-Forming & Proteolytic Bacteria

How Eggs Alter Gut Ecology

The gut microbiome responds rapidly to dietary input. Foods that digest cleanly favor carbohydrate-fermenting bacteria that produce short-chain fatty acids such as butyrate. Foods that resist digestion favor proteolytic and acid-forming species that generate toxic metabolites. Egg consumption consistently promotes the latter pattern.

Proteolytic bacteria metabolize amino acids into ammonia, hydrogen sulfide, phenols, and indoles. These compounds increase luminal toxicity and disrupt epithelial function. Hydrogen sulfide inhibits mitochondrial respiration in colonocytes, weakening barrier integrity and increasing permeability.

Eggs also increase systemic acid load. Sulfur-containing amino acids contribute to acid-forming residues that must be buffered through mineral withdrawal and renal excretion. Chronic acid burden promotes inflammation and contributes to bone and muscle catabolism over time.

As gut ecology shifts, beneficial species decline and opportunistic organisms expand. This imbalance, known as dysbiosis, creates a feedback loop in which digestion becomes progressively less efficient and inflammation becomes more persistent. Eggs help create this environment.

Lesson 7: Secondary Metabolites of Egg Digestion

Ammonia, Hydrogen Sulfide, Biogenic Amines, and Phenols

Secondary metabolites are compounds produced not by human cells, but by bacterial metabolism. When eggs are consumed, the secondary metabolites generated during fermentation exert direct toxic effects on intestinal and systemic health.

Ammonia damages epithelial cells and increases intestinal permeability. Biogenic amines such as putrescine and cadaverine disrupt cellular signaling and contribute to neuroinflammation. Phenols and indoles burden hepatic detoxification pathways and interfere with endocrine balance.

These compounds are absorbed into circulation, where they contribute to fatigue, brain fog, and inflammatory symptoms often attributed to unrelated causes. The issue is not acute poisoning, but chronic exposure to low-level toxins generated daily through digestion-resistant foods.

Eggs are particularly efficient at generating these compounds due to their protein density and lack of accompanying fiber. The absence of fermentable carbohydrates prevents dilution and buffering, intensifying toxicity.

Lesson 8: Endotoxins & Intestinal Permeability

Lipopolysaccharides, Inflammation, & Metabolic Endotoxemia

Endotoxins are inflammatory compounds derived from bacterial cell walls, particularly lipopolysaccharide. High-fat, digestion-resistant foods increase the absorption of these compounds from the gut into systemic circulation. Eggs contribute to this process through both their fat content and their promotion of dysbiosis.

When endotoxins enter the bloodstream, they activate immune pathways associated with insulin resistance, vascular dysfunction, and neuroinflammation. This state, known as metabolic endotoxemia, does not produce immediate illness but creates a chronic inflammatory baseline that accelerates disease progression.

Eggs exacerbate this process by slowing gastric emptying, impairing digestion, and increasing intestinal permeability. Over time, repeated endotoxin exposure contributes to the very conditions eggs are often claimed to prevent.

The gut is not merely a digestive organ. It is an immune interface. Foods that compromise its integrity compromise systemic health. Eggs, through their effects on digestion and microbial metabolism, consistently undermine that interface.

Part III: Fat, Cholesterol, & Metabolic Stress

While protein fermentation creates many of the immediate digestive consequences of egg consumption, fat and cholesterol drive many of the longer-term metabolic effects. Eggs are not merely a protein source. Each unit contains a concentrated package of saturated fat, dietary cholesterol, and lipid-soluble compounds that exert systemic influence far beyond the gut.

This section examines how egg-derived fats alter digestion, disrupt insulin signaling, damage vascular tissue, and accelerate metabolic disease. These effects are observable, measurable, and cumulative.

Lesson 9: Egg Fats & Delayed Gastric Emptying

How Fat Worsens Protein Fermentation

Egg yolks are dense in fat, with a composition heavily weighted toward saturated fatty acids. While fat is often framed as metabolically neutral or even beneficial in isolation, the presence significantly alters digestive dynamics. High-fat foods slow gastric emptying, keeping the stomach full longer before entering the small intestine.

This delay has important consequences for protein digestion. When digestion is slowed, enzymatic breakdown becomes less efficient. Proteins that are not fully hydrolyzed in the upper digestive tract are more likely to reach the colon intact, where they become substrate for bacterial fermentation rather than nourishment for human cells.

Egg fats exacerbate this problem by pairing digestion-resistant proteins with lipids that impair motility. The result is a digestive bottleneck that favors putrefaction over absorption. This process increases the production of ammonia, hydrogen sulfide, and other toxic metabolites discussed in the previous section.

Beyond digestion, high-fat meals stimulate the formation of chylomicrons, lipoprotein particles responsible for transporting dietary fat through the bloodstream. These particles have been shown to facilitate the absorption of bacterial endotoxins from the gut into circulation. In this way, egg fats act not only as a digestive burden, but as a delivery system for inflammatory compounds.

Repeated exposure to this pattern trains the body toward metabolic inefficiency. The digestive system becomes slower, microbial fermentation becomes more pronounced, and inflammatory signaling becomes more persistent. Eggs do not exist outside this context. Their fat content amplifies every digestive weakness they introduce.

Lesson 10: Dietary Cholesterol & Oxidative Injury

Oxysterols and Vascular Damage

Eggs are one of the most concentrated sources of dietary cholesterol in the modern diet. While cholesterol is an essential molecule synthesized endogenously by the human body, excess dietary cholesterol contributes to oxidative stress and vascular injury, particularly when consumed alongside saturated fat.

When dietary cholesterol is exposed to heat during cooking, the substance undergoes oxidation, forming compounds known as oxysterols. These cholesterol oxidation products are highly reactive and have been shown to damage endothelial cells, promote inflammation, and accelerate atherosclerotic plaque formation. Unlike native cholesterol, oxysterols are directly cytotoxic.

Even without cooking, excess dietary cholesterol increases the burden on hepatic lipid regulation. The liver must process, package, and redistribute cholesterol through lipoproteins, increasing circulating low-density lipoprotein particles. Elevated LDL particle number, rather than cholesterol concentration alone, is strongly associated with cardiovascular risk.

Egg-derived cholesterol also interacts with choline metabolism, contributing to the formation of trimethylamine oxide through microbial processing. TMAO has been identified as an independent risk factor for cardiovascular disease, promoting vascular inflammation.

The argument that dietary cholesterol does not matter because the body regulates our own synthesis overlooks the cumulative effects of repeated exposure. Regulation is not immunity. When excess input becomes routine, regulatory systems become strained, and damage accumulates silently.

Lesson 11: Pancreatic Load & Insulin Resistance

Intramyocellular Lipids & Glucose Dysregulation

The pancreas plays a central role in metabolic health, regulating blood glucose through insulin secretion. Diets high in saturated fat and dietary cholesterol place a disproportionate burden on this system, contributing to insulin resistance and beta-cell exhaustion over time. Eggs contribute to this burden in multiple ways.

Dietary fat increases the accumulation of lipids within muscle cells, a condition known as intramyocellular lipid deposition. These lipid droplets interfere with insulin signaling, preventing glucose from entering cells efficiently. As insulin sensitivity declines, the pancreas compensates by producing more insulin, creating a cycle of overproduction and eventual dysfunction.

Egg consumption has been consistently associated with increased risk of type 2 diabetes, particularly when intake is frequent. This association is not explained by calories alone. It reflects the combined effects of saturated fat, cholesterol, endotoxin absorption, and inflammatory signaling on insulin pathways.

Over time, pancreatic stress manifests as impaired glucose tolerance, elevated fasting insulin, and eventual beta-cell failure. Eggs are often promoted as a safe protein choice for blood sugar control, yet their metabolic effects directly undermine insulin sensitivity.

Insulin resistance does not develop overnight. It is the result of repeated metabolic insults that accumulate gradually. Eggs contribute to this process quietly, masked by their reputation as a benign food.

Part IV: Cooking, Denaturation, & Chemical Damage

Cooking is often framed as a solution to the problems associated with animal foods. Heat is said to improve digestibility, eliminate pathogens, and make nutrients more accessible. While cooking does neutralize certain bacterial risks, a separate and significant category of chemical damage is introduced, particularly when applied to foods already dense in fat and protein.

Eggs are uniquely vulnerable to heat-induced harm. Their combination of cholesterol, saturated fat, sulfur-containing amino acids, and glycation-prone proteins makes them a fertile substrate for oxidative injury and toxic compound formation. The effects of cooking eggs are not superficial. This process alters molecular structure, generates inflammatory byproducts, and accelerates biological aging.

This section examines what heat does to eggs at the chemical level, why cooked eggs are metabolically hostile, and how repeated exposure contributes to chronic disease processes.

Lesson 12: Protein Denaturation & Heat-Induced Toxicity

Structural Damage to Amino Acids

Protein denaturation refers to the alteration of a protein's three-dimensional structure under heat. While denaturation is often described as benign or even beneficial for digestion, this simplification ignores the downstream consequences of structural damage. When proteins are denatured, they lose not only their native shape but also their functional integrity.

Egg proteins are particularly sensitive to heat. Ovalbumin, ovotransferrin, and ovomucin undergo significant conformational changes when cooked. These changes expose reactive amino acid residues that are more prone to oxidation and glycation. Once altered, these proteins are more likely to provoke immune recognition, inflammation, and impaired digestion.

Cooking does not fully solve egg protein digestibility. While heat may reduce some enzyme inhibitors, this simultaneously creates new antigenic structures that are more difficult for the immune system to tolerate. This is one reason egg allergies and sensitivities persist even when eggs are thoroughly cooked.

Heat-damaged proteins also place a greater burden on detoxification pathways. The liver must process altered amino acids and nitrogenous waste products that would not be present if digestion were clean and efficient. Over time, this contributes to systemic inflammation & metabolic strain.

The narrative that cooked eggs are *"easier to digest"* obscures a critical distinction, that ease of digestion does not equal biological safety. A protein can be broken down more readily while still generating inflammatory signals and toxic intermediates. Cooking only changes the problem.

Lesson 13: Advanced Glycation End-Products

Accelerated Aging and Cellular Stress

Advanced glycation end-products, commonly referred to as AGEs, are compounds formed when proteins or fats bind to sugars under heat. While AGEs can form endogenously, dietary AGEs represent a significant and often overlooked source of oxidative stress. When cooked, eggs become a concentrated source of these compounds.

Egg proteins readily undergo glycation due to their amino acid composition and exposure to heat. The presence of fat further accelerates AGE formation. Once ingested, dietary AGEs bind to receptors known as RAGE (receptors for advanced glycation end-products), activating inflammatory pathways throughout the body.

AGE accumulation has been linked to endothelial dysfunction, kidney disease, neurodegeneration, and accelerated skin aging. These compounds also shorten telomeres, contributing to premature cellular senescence. Importantly, AGEs are not efficiently cleared by the body. Repeated exposure leads to more accumulation.

Individuals with diabetes, insulin resistance, or compromised kidney function are particularly vulnerable to AGE burden. Despite this vulnerability, eggs are often recommended to these populations as a "safe" protein source, compounding the conditions they intend to manage.

AGE formation is not an unavoidable consequence of eating. This is strongly influenced by food choice and preparation. Diets centered on whole plant foods generate far fewer AGEs than those rich in cooked animal products. Eggs, due to their structure and cooking methods, consistently rank among the highest AGE contributors per serving.

Lesson 14: Neu5Gc, Sialic Acid Binding, & Immune Activation

Why Egg Proteins Provoke Chronic Inflammation

Neu5Gc is a sialic acid found in many animal-derived foods but not produced naturally by the human body. When consumed, Neu5Gc becomes incorporated into human tissues, and is then recognized as foreign by the immune system. This creates a state of chronic, low-grade inflammation described as *"xenosialitis."*

Eggs contribute to this process through glycoproteins that bind sialic acids and facilitate immune recognition. When egg proteins are cooked and denatured, their antigenicity increases, enhancing immune activation. This is particularly relevant for individuals with autoimmune conditions, allergies, or compromised gut barriers.

The immune system does not distinguish between "small" and "large" inflammatory signals. Chronic exposure to antigenic compounds keeps immune pathways activated, diverting resources away from tissue repair and increasing disease susceptibility. Over time, this immune burden contributes to systemic inflammation, endothelial dysfunction, and cancer risk.

The inflammatory effects of Neu5Gc are subtle but persistent. Unlike acute allergic reactions, xenosialitis operates quietly, shaping disease risk over years rather than days. Eggs, by repeatedly introducing foreign sialic acid structures, participate in this slow-burning inflammatory process.

Understanding immune activation requires moving beyond symptom-based thinking. Foods do not need to cause immediate reactions to be harmful. They only need to create sustained immune engagement. Eggs do this reliably.

Part V: Eggs, Disease, & Long-Term Risk

Digestive distress and metabolic strain are often dismissed as short-term inconveniences, but their true significance lies in what they initiate over time. Chronic inflammation, insulin resistance, endothelial dysfunction, and immune activation do not arise suddenly. They develop through repeated exposures that quietly shift physiology away from balance and toward disease.

Egg consumption has been consistently associated with increased risk of multiple chronic conditions. These associations persist across populations, study designs, and decades of research. While correlation alone does not prove causation, the convergence of epidemiological data with known biological mechanisms strengthens the case considerably.

This section examines the relationship between egg consumption and long-term disease risk, integrating population-level findings with the digestive, metabolic, and inflammatory pathways explored in earlier chapters.

Lesson 15: Egg Consumption & Cardiovascular Disease

Atherosclerosis, Coronary Calcium, & Stroke

Cardiovascular disease remains the leading cause of death worldwide. While genetics play a role, the dominant drivers of vascular disease are dietary and metabolic. Eggs have long been positioned as neutral or even protective within this context, despite their cholesterol content and fat composition. Population data tells a different story.

Multiple cohort studies have identified a dose-dependent relationship between egg consumption and cardiovascular risk. Increased intake correlates with higher incidence of coronary artery disease, greater coronary artery calcium scores, and elevated stroke risk. These findings are particularly pronounced among individuals with insulin resistance or diabetes, suggesting metabolic vulnerability amplifies egg-related harm.

Coronary artery calcium scoring provides a direct measure of atherosclerotic burden. Studies have demonstrated that individuals who consume eggs frequently exhibit significantly higher calcium scores than those who avoid eggs, even after adjusting for lifestyle factors. Calcium deposition reflects cumulative vascular injury rather than short-term fluctuation, making this association especially concerning.

Mechanistically, egg-derived cholesterol contributes to endothelial dysfunction through oxidative modification of lipoproteins. Oxidized LDL particles infiltrate arterial walls, triggering inflammatory cascades and foam cell formation. Over time, these processes lead to plaque development and arterial stiffening. Egg-related increases in TMAO further exacerbate vascular inflammation and thrombosis risk.

Stroke risk follows a similar pattern. Hemorrhagic and ischemic strokes are both influenced by endothelial integrity, blood viscosity, and inflammatory tone. Egg consumption has been associated with increased stroke incidence, particularly hemorrhagic stroke, likely due to combined effects on blood pressure regulation, vascular fragility, and clotting pathways.

The claim that eggs are heart-healthy relies on selective interpretation of short-term lipid markers rather than long-term outcomes. When viewed across decades rather than weeks, the cardiovascular cost of egg consumption becomes difficult to ignore.

Lesson 16: Eggs & Diabetes

Meta-Analyses, Mechanisms, & Pancreatic Exhaustion

Type II diabetes is a disease of metabolic overload that develops when insulin signaling is chronically impaired by lipid accumulation, inflammation, and oxidative stress. Eggs contribute to each of these processes, making their association with diabetes biologically plausible and repeatedly observable.

Large prospective cohort studies have found that individuals who consume the most eggs experience significantly higher rates of type II diabetes than those who consume few or none. Meta-analyses incorporating hundreds of thousands of participants confirm this association, particularly in Western populations where eggs are consumed alongside high-fat diets.

The pancreas responds to insulin resistance by increasing insulin output. Over time, this compensatory mechanism fails, leading to beta-cell dysfunction. Egg consumption accelerates this process by increasing intramyocellular lipid accumulation, endotoxin absorption, and inflammatory signaling. Each of these factors impairs insulin receptor sensitivity.

Egg-derived AGEs further burden pancreatic tissue. AGE accumulation has been shown to damage beta cells directly and worsen glycemic control. Additionally, chronic exposure to dietary cholesterol disrupts membrane fluidity in insulin-sensitive tissues, impairing glucose uptake.

Notably, the increased diabetes risk associated with egg consumption persists even after adjusting for body weight. This indicates that the effect is not merely caloric, but mechanistic. Eggs interfere with glucose regulation in ways that extend beyond energy balance.

Recommending eggs as a diabetes-friendly food ignores this evidence and misrepresents metabolic reality. For individuals at risk of insulin resistance, eggs represent an avoidable burden rather than a protective nutrient.

Lesson 17: Eggs & Cancer Risk

Breast Cancer, Prostate Cancer, & Hormonal Pathways

Cancer development is influenced by growth signaling, inflammation, and immune surveillance. Eggs interact with all three. Their protein content stimulates IGF-1, their fats promote oxidative stress, and their choline and androgen content influence hormone-sensitive tissues.

Epidemiological studies have identified strong correlations between egg consumption and increased risk of breast and prostate cancers. Women consuming more than half an egg per day have been shown to experience significantly higher breast cancer incidence. Men consuming multiple eggs per week exhibit elevated risk of lethal prostate cancer.

Choline metabolism plays a central role in this association. Animal-derived choline is metabolized into TMAO, which has been linked to cancer progression and metastasis. Eggs are among the richest sources of choline in the diet, compounding exposure.

Egg yolks also contain androgenic compounds that influence prostate tissue growth. Chronic stimulation of androgen receptors increases proliferation risk and may accelerate tumor development. Combined with inflammatory signaling and immune distraction, this creates a permissive environment for malignancy.

Cancer emerges from sustained biological conditions that favor growth over regulation. Eggs contribute to these conditions quietly and consistently, masked by their reputation as benign.

Lesson 18: Eggs and Longevity

Competing Risk Analysis and Mortality Data

Longevity research evaluates not just whether people live longer, but how dietary choices influence disease burden over time. Competing risk analysis allows researchers to compare the impact of different behaviors on mortality. Within this framework, egg consumption consistently performs poorly.

Long-term cohort studies have demonstrated that daily egg consumption shortens lifespan by increasing cumulative cardiovascular and metabolic risk. In some analyses, the cholesterol burden from one egg per day has been compared to the mortality impact of smoking multiple cigarettes daily over extended periods.

These findings do not imply equivalence of harm, but they underscore proportional risk. Eggs exert a measurable toll on longevity through mechanisms that compound slowly such as vascular injury, insulin resistance, immune activation, and oxidative stress.

Longevity is not extended by single nutrients, but by reducing cumulative biological insults. Eggs add to that burden without providing compensatory benefits unavailable from safer sources. When evaluated through the lens of lifespan rather than convenience, eggs fail the test of long-term nourishment.

Part VI: Immunity, Viruses, & Chronic Illness

The immune system can be perceived as a form of communication that listens constantly to food, microbes, memory, stress, and the subtle signals carried through the gut and bloodstream. Our immunity learns through relationship, not domination. When nourishment is coherent, the immune system rests into discernment. When nourishment is confused, the immune system never sleeps.

Modern illness is not defined by the presence of pathogens alone but is defined by immune exhaustion after the system is asked to respond endlessly to signals that do not belong. Eggs, though rarely accused, participate in this confusion. Not dramatically, but quietly and persistently.

This section explores how egg consumption influences immune signaling, viral behavior, and chronic inflammatory states. The information is not presented through a lens of fear, but through a sense of deep understanding.

Lesson 19: Eggs as Viral Growth Media

When Nourishment Feeds the Wrong Life

Viruses do not eat the way humans do. They do not digest fiber or metabolize glucose for energy. They rely on host machinery and available substrates to replicate. Certain proteins, lipids, and growth-promoting compounds accelerate this process. Eggs, by their very nature, are designed to support rapid biological expansion.

For decades, the vaccine industry has relied on egg allantois tissue to culture viruses, particularly influenza strains. This practice is not incidental. Egg proteins provide an ideal environment for viral replication. The same qualities that support embryonic development, such as dense amino acids, growth signaling, and lipid scaffolding, also support viral proliferation.

This raises an uncomfortable but necessary question. If eggs are known to facilitate viral growth in laboratory settings, how might they influence viral behavior within the human body?

Emerging research suggests that exposure to egg-derived proteins can provoke immune responses unrelated to the targeted pathogen. Studies have documented antibody formation against egg-specific sugars, such as N-acetyllactosamine, rather than against viral antigens. This phenomenon reflects immune misdirection, where a system is responding vigorously, but not accurately.

Chronic viral presence is increasingly recognized as a contributing factor in fatigue syndromes, autoimmune conditions, neurological disorders, and inflammatory disease. Viruses such as Epstein–Barr, cytomegalovirus, and herpes family viruses persist latently within tissues, reactivating under conditions of immune stress.

Foods that promote inflammation or growth signaling may quietly support this reactivation. This does not imply that eggs introduce viruses but suggests that they may influence the internal environment in which viruses behave. Immunity is not only about defense but also about terrain. When the terrain favors expansion rather than regulation, balance is lost.

Lesson 20: Immune Confusion & Molecular Mimicry

When the Body Cannot Tell Friend from Foe

The immune system learns by pattern recognition. Self from non-self is distinguished through subtle molecular signatures. When those signatures overlap and foreign compounds resemble human tissue, the immune system becomes uncertain. This phenomenon is known as molecular mimicry.

Egg proteins contain structures that can resemble components of human tissue, particularly when denatured through cooking or partially digested in the gut. When these proteins cross a compromised intestinal barrier, they may be flagged as threats. Over time, repeated exposure trains the immune system toward hypervigilance.

Hypervigilance equates to exhaustion. An immune system locked in constant alert loses nuance. Inflammatory responses become broader, less precise, and more damaging. Autoimmune patterns emerge not because the body turns against itself, but because our system can no longer clearly perceive what belongs.

Inflammation driven by dietary antigens is subtle and does not announce itself as an allergy but whispers through joint stiffness, brain fog, sinus congestion, skin eruptions, and chronic fatigue. These signals are often dismissed as stress or aging. Truth is, they reflect an immune system struggling to resolve confusion.

When food ceases to provoke immune engagement, clarity returns. The immune system then remembers discernment and rest becomes possible again.

Lesson 21: Egg Proteins, Chronic Inflammation, & Immune Fatigue

The Cost of Never Fully Resting

Inflammation is a tool of repair and is not inherently harmful. When this condition becomes chronic, however, repair gives way to depletion. The immune system then expends energy without resolution, healing stalls, and fatigue deepens.

Egg consumption contributes to this pattern by repeatedly activating immune pathways through digestion-resistant proteins, endotoxin absorption, and antigenic exposure. While each exposure is small, together, they form a constant background hum of immune activation.

Chronic inflammation alters hormonal signaling, disrupts sleep architecture, and impairs mitochondrial energy production. This creates a state in which the body feels under siege even in the absence of immediate threat. Many modern illnesses are not the result of attack, but of exhaustion.

When eggs are removed from the diet, many individuals report a gradual softening of symptoms. There is significantly less congestion, clearer thinking, improved energy, and fewer inflammatory flares. This is a sign of relief, not placebo. The immune system is no longer asked to respond to a stimulus that does not belong.

Health requires rhythm, not constant stimulation. The immune system, like the nervous system, heals in moments of quiet. Foods that provoke without nourishing steal that quiet away.

Part VII: Clinical Pattern Recognition

Disease often arrives as a pattern and rarely is announced loudly in beginning stages. This can be experienced at first as a heaviness that does not lift, digestion that feels burdened rather than nourished, or a mind that clouds before breaks.

The body speaks long before collapse. Modern medicine often listens only when the language becomes extreme. This section listens earlier and traces the recurring clinical patterns that emerge when eggs remain in the diet. These are not perceived as isolated symptoms, but as relationships between systems.

Pattern recognition is an ancient skill that aligns with how healers once learned. This describes how the body remembers balance. When certain foods repeatedly precede the same clusters of symptoms, the signal becomes difficult to ignore. Eggs reveal themselves clearly when we learn how to listen.

Lesson 22: What Egg Sensitivity Actually Looks Like

Digestive, Neurological, & Inflammatory Patterns

Egg sensitivity does not usually arrive as anaphylaxis or immediate reaction. Instead, the accumulation unfolds quietly through digestion, skin, mood, and energy. Many individuals who tolerate eggs well in childhood begin to experience subtle intolerance as adults, particularly as digestive efficiency declines.

Digestively, egg sensitivity often presents as bloating, sluggish transit, sulfurous gas, or alternating constipation and loose stools. These symptoms reflect protein fermentation and bile stress rather than acute allergy. The absence of pain is frequently misinterpreted as tolerance, even as inflammation quietly increases.

Neurologically, eggs are associated with brain fog, irritability, anxiety, and difficulty concentrating. These effects are often attributed to stress or sleep deprivation, yet they frequently improve when eggs are removed. Endotoxin absorption, inflammatory cytokines, and biogenic amines all influence neurotransmitter balance and neural clarity.

Inflammatory patterns include sinus congestion, postnasal drip, joint stiffness, skin eruptions, and flare-ups of autoimmune conditions. These symptoms reflect immune activation rather than infection. Eggs do not cause these conditions directly, but they aggravate terrain in which inflammation already seeks expression.

The most revealing aspect of egg sensitivity is the reversibility. When eggs are removed, symptoms often soften within weeks. Digestion lightens, mental clarity returns, and inflammation recedes. These changes are not sudden miracles. They are the body remembering coherence.

Lesson 23: Why People Feel "Fine" Until They Don't

Latency, Compensation, & Metabolic Masking

The human body is extraordinarily adaptive and compensates long before failing. This capacity allows people to feel functional even as imbalance accumulates. Egg-related stress often operates within this window of compensation, where symptoms are muted and warnings are subtle.

The pancreas produces more insulin. The liver increases detoxification. The immune system tolerates antigenic load. The nervous system dampens inflammatory signals. These adaptations preserve outward stability, but they consume internal reserves.

Eggs contribute to this depletion through cumulative burden rather than acute harm. Saturated fat impairs insulin signaling gradually. Endotoxins inflame quietly. AGEs accumulate without sensation. Immune vigilance becomes constant background noise. None of this feels urgent until capacity is exceeded.

This is why people often defend foods that are harming them. "I feel fine" becomes evidence of safety. Feeling fine, though, is not the same as being aligned. By the time symptoms become undeniable, appearing as diabetes, autoimmune disease, or cardiovascular events, the underlying pattern has been present for years.

Clinical wisdom lies in noticing what the body has been compensating for. Removing eggs often reveals this truth gently. Energy returns not because something new was added, but because something burdensome was finally removed.

Lesson 24: Eggs in Children, Hormonal Development, & Neuroinflammation

Early Exposure and Lifelong Patterning

Children are not small adults. Their nervous systems, immune systems, and endocrine pathways are actively forming. Foods consumed during development influence not only growth, but regulatory tone. This is the baseline from which the body learns what is normal.

Eggs are often introduced early due to their soft texture and protein content. Yet early exposure to antigenic proteins can shape immune reactivity for years. Pediatric eczema, food sensitivities, asthma, and behavioral symptoms frequently correlate with early dietary triggers that were never identified.

Hormonal development is particularly sensitive to dietary fat and cholesterol. Excessive exposure to animal-derived lipids influences steroid hormone synthesis and insulin signaling during critical windows of growth. These influences do not create immediate disease, but they shape susceptibility.

Neuroinflammation during development alters attention, mood regulation, and stress response. Emerging research highlights the role of gut-derived inflammation in conditions such as ADHD, anxiety, and sensory sensitivity. Eggs, through their effects on digestion and immune signaling, may quietly contribute to these patterns in vulnerable children.

Nourishment during childhood should support clarity, resilience, and growth without burden. Removing eggs from children's diets often creates calm, not deficiency.

Part VIII: Comparative Risk Synthesis

Understanding harm requires comparison. Not to excuse one burden by pointing to another, but to recognize patterns of stress across systems.

Eggs are often defended by contrast. They are considered less harmful than meat, cleaner than dairy, and simpler than processed foods. Harm, however, is not erased by relativity. Biology responds to cumulative pressure, repeated exposure, and subtle disruption and does not grade on a curve.

This section places eggs beside meat and dairy, not to collapse them into sameness, but to clarify how each burdens the body differently. Only through comparison does the unique signature of egg consumption become fully visible.

Lesson 25: Eggs vs Meat vs Dairy

Different Foods, Different Burdens

Meat, dairy, and eggs are often grouped together as animal products, yet their physiological impacts are distinct. Each interacts with digestion, metabolism, immunity, and hormonal signaling in a characteristic way. Understanding these differences reveals why eggs are often underestimated.

Meat exerts the greatest strain through density. Large quantities of animal muscle tissue introduce heavy protein loads, heme iron, and inflammatory lipids that challenge digestion and increase oxidative stress. The burden is often felt quickly through heaviness, fatigue, and digestive discomfort. Meat's effects are blunt and noticeable.

Dairy exerts influence hormonally and immunologically. Casein proteins resist digestion and frequently provoke immune reactivity. Lactose challenges metabolic tolerance. Hormones intended to stimulate growth in calves influence human endocrine systems. Dairy's impact often appears through mucus production, skin conditions, sinus congestion, and inflammatory disease.

Eggs operate differently. They are smaller, lighter, and easier to justify. Their harm is not immediate heaviness or overt reaction, but subtle penetration. Eggs concentrate reproductive signaling, cholesterol, and antigenic proteins into a compact form that slips beneath awareness. Their effects accumulate quietly through daily exposure rather than dramatic episodes.

Each food burdens a different system most heavily. Meat stresses digestion and oxidation. Dairy stresses immunity and hormones. Eggs stress metabolism, immunity, and vascular integrity simultaneously. This overlap makes eggs uniquely deceptive. They rarely cause immediate distress, yet they quietly erode resilience over time.

Understanding this distinction dissolves the false hierarchy of "least bad." Health is not about choosing the lesser burden. The choice must remain coherence.

Lesson 26: Why Eggs Appeared Safer Than They Were

Invisibility, Frequency, & Cultural Blindness

Eggs escaped scrutiny not because they were harmless, but because their effects were diffused. They rarely triggered dramatic symptoms. They were eaten in small quantities and embedded in routine. This made their influence difficult to isolate.

Unlike meat, eggs do not overwhelm digestion immediately. Unlike dairy, they do not always produce visible mucus or skin reactions. Their harm unfolds beneath perception, through lipid accumulation, immune activation, and metabolic stress that progress silently.

Frequency plays a decisive role. Eggs are rarely eaten occasionally. They are eaten daily. The body tolerates occasional stress and struggles under constant repetition. A food consumed every morning becomes part of baseline physiology. The effects are then mistaken for normal aging, normal fatigue, and normal decline.

Cultural reinforcement further obscured the signal. Eggs were marketed as virtuous for being protein-rich, affordable, and disciplined. Questioning them felt unnecessary and even ungrateful. Over time, this cultural protection insulated eggs from reevaluation, even as evidence accumulated.

Invisibility, however, is not innocence and is often the most dangerous form of harm.

Lesson 27: Frequency Matters More Than Quantity

The Quiet Weight of Repetition

The body is remarkably forgiving and can recover from indulgence, missteps, and short-term excess. What we cannot easily recover from is repetition. Small insults repeated daily accumulate into systemic strain.

Eggs exemplify this principle. One egg may not produce noticeable harm. Two eggs may feel benign. Yet when consumed daily over years, their metabolic effects compound. Cholesterol accumulates, while lipids infiltrate muscle tissue, immune activation becomes chronic, and endotoxin exposure becomes routine.

This pattern explains why many people defend eggs passionately. The harm does not announce itself dramatically, but whispers through gradual fatigue, creeping insulin resistance, subtle inflammation, and declining clarity. By the time disease manifests, the original cause feels distant.

Health is not lost through singular choices but is shaped through rhythm. Foods eaten daily shape baseline physiology. Foods eaten occasionally do not. Removing eggs from daily rotation often produces disproportionate benefit. This is not because eggs are uniquely toxic, but because repetition amplifies their effects.

Wisdom lies not in moderation alone, but in discernment. The body remembers what we are asked to process repeatedly and adapts for as long as possible.

Part IX: Transitioning Without Deficiency

The fear that arises when a familiar food is questioned is rarely about the food itself and is often more about survival. Will I have enough? Will my body weaken? Will something essential be lost?

These fears deserve tenderness, not dismissal. The body remembers famine more clearly than abundance, yet nourishment is not created by holding tightly to what burdens us. Our health is restored when the body is allowed to breathe again.

This section is not about substitution for the sake of mimicry but is about restoring biological coherence by meeting nutritional needs without provoking inflammation, fermentation, or immune fatigue.

Lesson 28: Protein Without Putrefaction

Amino Acids That Build Without Burden

Protein acquisition has been misunderstood as a singular substance rather than a biological process. The body does not require protein in the form of the food that appears on a plate. We require amino acids, and the raw materials that are assembled as needed, where needed, and when needed.

Whole plant foods provide amino acids in a form that supports digestion rather than overwhelms. When amino acids arrive bound to fiber, water, and phytonutrients, they are absorbed gradually in the small intestine, reducing fermentation and endotoxin production. This delivery system honors the body's pace.

Greens, legumes, seeds, nuts, fruits, and sea vegetables all contribute to the amino acid pool. No single food must carry the burden alone. Variety creates sufficiency and balance creates utilization. The myth that strength requires density collapses when digestion is efficient and inflammation is low.

Removing eggs often improves protein utilization rather than diminishing. When the gut is no longer burdened by digestion-resistant proteins, assimilation improves. Energy increases not because more protein is consumed, but because less is wasted in fermentation and immune response.

Protein that builds without putrefaction restores confidence. The body recognizes nourishment when we do not have to defend ourselves from what we ingest.

Lesson 29: Choline, Biotin, & the Myth of Nutrient Dependence

Abundance Without Concentration

Eggs are often defended based on specific nutrients, and particularly choline and biotin. This defense assumes that nutrients are scarce and must be obtained in concentrated form. Biology tells a different story.

Choline is abundant throughout the plant kingdoms and queendoms. Cruciferous vegetables, legumes, seeds, and leafy greens provide choline in forms that do not promote TMAO formation. When choline is delivered alongside fiber and antioxidants, the vitamin supports cellular function without provoking vascular inflammation.

Biotin, similarly, is widely available in fruits, seeds, nuts, and vegetables. Unlike egg-derived biotin, plant-based sources are not bound to avidin. For this reason, absorption proceeds unimpeded. Utilization then improves when the gut is no longer inflamed or compromised.

The body requires accessibility, not nutrient concentration. When digestion is clear and the microbiome is balanced, micronutrient sufficiency follows naturally. Removing eggs often reveals this truth quickly, as hair, skin, and energy improve rather than decline.

Nutrient myths persist because they simplify complexity, but nourishment is a relationship, not a checklist.

Lesson 30: Satiety, Strength, & Sustained Energy

Why Fullness Should Feel Light

True satiety feels calm, clear, and stable. Nutritional fulfillment does not demand rest after eating or cloud the mind. Eggs are often praised for their ability to create fullness, yet that fullness frequently arises from delayed digestion rather than nourishment.

Plant-based meals create satiety through volume, fiber, hydration, and micronutrient sufficiency. Blood sugar stabilizes gently, while energy remains accessible, and the nervous system does not enter defensive mode. This form of fullness supports movement rather than discouraging.

Strength follows clarity. Muscles recover more efficiently when inflammation is low and circulation is unobstructed. Endurance improves when mitochondria are not burdened by oxidative stress and lipid overload. Removing eggs often reveals this shift within weeks, particularly in individuals engaged in physical training or endurance activity.

Sustained energy is not extracted from food through force, and emerges when the body is not fighting digestion, immune activation, or endotoxin exposure. Foods that nourish without provoking allow energy to flow rather than spike and crash. When satiety feels light, strength becomes sustainable.

Part X: Philosophical Integration

We could feel when our body was nourished long before we began measuring nutrition. Before calories were counted, the body listened. Before food became commodity, we forged relationship with our meals.

Modern illness is not simply the result of wrong information but is the result of forgetting how to listen. Biology still speaks clearly yet now speaks softly. When habit becomes louder than sensation, nourishment loses way. This section returns to first principles to place science back into relationship with wisdom.

Lesson 31: Reproductive Foods & Evolutionary Confusion

When Growth Signals Outlive Their Purpose

Every food carries intention that is rooted in biological purpose. Seeds are intended to sprout, fruits are meant to be eaten, leaves are to be browsed, and eggs hatch as life.

When reproductive material is consumed regularly by a species not designed to receive these codes, confusion arises. Growth signals persist beyond their context, and the body receives messages intended for embryonic expansion rather than long-term maintenance.

Evolution favors efficiency, not excess. Human physiology evolved around foods that ripen, decay, and regenerate in rhythm with the seasons. Reproductive tissues from another species were never meant to become daily staples. Their modern abundance is an anomaly, not an adaptation, and the result of factory farming, mass breeding, and often artificial insemination.

This confusion is expressed subtly. Cells receive signals to grow when they should repair. Hormones stimulate when they are expected to rest. Immunity remains alert rather than naturally softening. Disease emerges not as punishment, but as miscommunication sustained over time.

When foods align with evolutionary rhythm, clarity returns. Our body remembers the original instructions.

Lesson 32: When Culture Replaces Listening

Habit, Authority, & The Silencing of the Body

Culture teaches us what to ignore. When a food is eaten by everyone, effects disappear into the background. Discomfort then becomes normal, fatigue becomes age, and inflammation becomes inevitability. Culture reassures us that nothing is wrong because nothing is questioned.

Authority reinforces this silence. Institutions speak in averages, while the body requires particulars. When lived experience contradicts guidance, experience is often dismissed. The body never lies, though, and compensates, adapts, and signals until the load can no longer be carried.

Listening requires humility. We must acknowledge that tradition may persist beyond usefulness. We are releasing identity from habit. When eggs are removed from the diet and clarity returns, the body offers evidence that is quiet, undeniable, and personal. Health comes from relationship, not obedience.

Lesson 33: Food as Relationship, Not Commodity

Returning to Coherence

To eat is to enter relationship with land, time, and the unseen labor of growth and decay. When food becomes commodity, this relationship collapses into transaction. The body receives calories but not coherence.

Foods that nourish without burden invite presence. Digestion becomes quiet, energy steadies, and thought clears. These changes are gentle and not dramatic. Healing arrives as relief and rarely shouts.

Removing eggs is an act of discernment, not an act of rejection. We are choosing foods that speak the body's language fluently, and honoring metabolism as a sacred conversation rather than a machine to be forced.

When nourishment is aligned, restraint dissolves. Choice then becomes intuitive and the body remembers how to guide itself. The way has always known. We simply learn again how to listen.

Part XI: Summary, Clarity, & Closure

Truth does not demand agreement but waits to be seen. By the time the body understands something fully, the tension as often already resolved and the concept feels obvious. This generally ends the argument. What remains is a sense of alignment and a quiet recognition that something unnecessary has been released.

This final section gathers what has been revealed, not to persuade further, but to clarify what is already present.

Lesson 34: What the Evidence Actually Says

A Clear Accounting

Across many disciplines, including nutrition science, epidemiology, immunology, and clinical observation, the story of egg consumption is remarkably consistent. Eggs are not essential, or protective, and clearly are not benign.

The evidence does not point to a single catastrophic outcome, but to cumulative burden. Eggs impair digestion through protein resistance and fermentation. They strain metabolism through saturated fat and cholesterol. They activate immune pathways through antigenic proteins and endotoxin absorption. Over time, these pressures converge into increased risk for cardiovascular disease, diabetes, cancer, immune dysfunction, and premature aging.

Equally important is what the evidence does not show. There is no unique nutrient in eggs that cannot be obtained safely elsewhere. There is no population that requires eggs for optimal health. There is no long-term data demonstrating protective effects independent of confounding lifestyle factors.

When stripped of marketing language and cultural attachment, the scientific record becomes clear. Eggs persist in the diet not because they serve human biology well, but because they have been normalized beyond question.

Lesson 35: Who Should Most Avoid Eggs

Listening to Vulnerability

While eggs impose measurable burden on the general population, certain individuals are particularly susceptible to their effects. Vulnerability does not imply weakness but reflects genetic, metabolic, and environmental context.

Those with insulin resistance, diabetes, or a family history of metabolic disease are among the most affected. Eggs exacerbate lipid accumulation and inflammatory signaling that undermine glucose regulation. For these individuals, removing eggs often produces noticeable improvements in energy and glycemic stability.

Individuals with autoimmune conditions, chronic fatigue, neurological symptoms, or digestive disorders also tend to respond strongly. In these cases, eggs act less as nourishment and more as noise, continually provoking immune engagement that prevents resolution.

Children deserve special consideration. Developing immune systems and nervous systems are more impressionable. Foods that provoke inflammation or antigenic stress during development can shape long-term sensitivity. Nourishment in childhood should reduce burden, not introduce harm.

Nothing presented in this book circulates around fear. We present information with accuracy and gentleness. When vulnerability is honored, healing becomes more likely.

Lesson 36: A Return to Coherence

Letting the Body Lead

Healing requires removal of what obstructs. When eggs are no longer present, the body does not struggle to compensate and can rest peacefully. Digestion also quiets, while immunity recalibrates, and energy returns without demand.

This return is subtle and deeply familiar. Many people describe the feeling as being "more themselves." That phrase is telling. The body was burdened but never broken.

To release eggs is not to adopt an identity but to practice discernment. We decide to choose foods that do not require defense and allow nourishment to feel like clarity rather than effort. The body knows how to heal if not interrupted. The way has always known.

Appendices

Appendix A: Beyond the Egg

Whole-Food, Oil-Free, Plant-Based Alternatives

The recipes that follow avoid refined oils, isolated flavor enhancers, and processed binders. Heat is applied gently where necessary, and water-based or dry-heat cooking methods are favored. The goal is not to imitate eggs, but to replace the functional binding, structure, and nourishment without introducing biological interference.

Eggs were never essential to human vitality, only habitual. When digestion is honored and the microbiome is supported, nourishment becomes effortless rather than demanding. These foods do not mimic the egg. They surpass the egg nutritionally by aligning with the body rather than challenging our biological processes.

1. Chickpea Morning Cake (Egg-Free Omelet Alternative)

Free From: Eggs, Soy, Grains, Oils, Alliums

Ingredients

- 1 cup chickpea flour
- ½ cup sun-dried tomatoes
- ¾ cup filtered water
- ¼ teaspoon turmeric
- Black pepper, smoked paprika, oregano & red Alaea sea salt

Optional Fillers

- Finely crumbled Pum-Fu, Steamed Spinach, Sweet Potatoes, Diced Heirloom Tomatoes & Sliced Avocado

Preparation

1. In a Vitamix or high-powered blender, mix all ingredients.
2. Preheat a non-stick (PFAS free) or well-seasoned ceramic pan over medium-low heat.
3. Pour batter into pan and spread evenly.
4. Cook 4–5 minutes until edges lift easily.
5. Flip gently and cook another 3 minutes until set.
6. Add fillers
7. Serve warm or cooled.

2. Pumpkin Seed Breakfast Scramble

Free From: Eggs, Soy, Grains, Oils, Alliums

Ingredients

- 1 cup raw pumpkin seeds
- ½ cup chopped summer squash
- 1 bunch cilantro
- ¼ teaspoon turmeric
- Splash filtered water

Preparation

1. Soak pumpkin seeds in water for 6-8 hours, then drain.
2. Pulse soaked seeds in a food processor until coarse and crumb-like.
3. Add zucchini and turmeric, then pulse briefly.
4. Transfer to a dry skillet over medium heat.
5. Add a splash of water to prevent sticking.
6. Stir continuously for 5–7 minutes until warmed and slightly firm.
7. Remove from heat and rest 2 minutes before serving.
8. Add chopped cilantro to the dish before serving.
9. Season after removed from heat with red Alaea sea salt, Black Pepper, Smoked Paprika, Chipotle Powder, & Oregano.

3. Golden Mung Bean Cakes

Free From: Eggs, Soy, Grains, Oils, Alliums

Ingredients

- 1 cup dried mung beans
- ¼ teaspoon turmeric
- 1 tablespoon ground flaxseed or chia seed powder
- 3 tablespoons water

Preparation

1. Soak mung beans overnight; drain and rinse.
2. Blend beans with turmeric and enough water to form thick batter.
3. Mix flaxseed or chia with water separately to form gel, then fold into batter.
4. Preheat non-stick or ceramic pan over medium-low heat.
5. Spoon batter into small cakes.
6. Cook 4 minutes per side until lightly browned and firm.
7. Allow to cool slightly before serving.

4. Chia–Hemp Protein Custard (No Heat Option)

Free From: Eggs, Soy, Grains, Oils, Alliums

Ingredients

- 2 tablespoons chia seeds
- 2 tablespoons hemp seeds
- 1 cup coconut milk or almond milk
- 4 pitted, then chopped dates
- ¼ teaspoon Ceylon cinnamon
- Optional vanilla bean powder or scrapings

Preparation

1. Combine all ingredients in glass jar or bowl.
2. Stir thoroughly to prevent clumping.
3. Cover and refrigerate at least 4 hours or overnight.
4. Stir again before serving.

5. Socca-Style Chickpea Flatbread (Oil-Free)

Free From: Eggs, Soy, Grains, Oils, Alliums

Ingredients

- 1 cup chickpea flour
- 1 cup water
- Pinch red Alaea salt (optional)
- Optional dried herbs (Basil, Cilantro, Rosemary, Sage or Thyme)

Preparation

1. Whisk flour and water until smooth.
2. Let batter rest 30 minutes.
3. Preheat oven to 425°F (220°C).
4. Pour batter into parchment-lined baking dish.
5. Bake 15–20 minutes until firm and lightly golden.
6. Cool before slicing.

6. Pum-Fu Morning Hash (Optional Inclusion)

Note: Pum-Fu is pumpkin-seed-based and not soy.

Ingredients

- ½ block Pum-Fu, crumbled
- 1 cup diced sweet potato
- ½ cup bell pepper
- Splash water

Preparation

1. Steam sweet potato until just tender.
2. Add potatoes, pepper, and Pum-Fu to pan over medium heat.
3. Add water as needed to prevent sticking.
4. Stir and warm 6–8 minutes.
5. Add seasonings (black pepper, chipotle powder, cumin, oregano, red Alaea sea salt and smoked paprika) after removed from heat.
6. Serve immediately.

7. Flax–Almond Binding Gel (Egg Replacement)

Use: Baking, patties, structure

Ingredients

- 1 tablespoon ground flaxseed
- 1 tablespoon almond flour
- 3 tablespoons warm water

Preparation

1. Mix all ingredients in small bowl.
2. Let sit 5 minutes until gel forms.
3. Use immediately as egg replacement.

Appendix B: Biological Mechanisms by Body System

Egg consumption affects the human body through multiple overlapping systems. While individual chapters explore these effects in detail, this appendix provides a consolidated overview of the primary mechanisms involved.

Digestive System

Egg proteins resist complete enzymatic breakdown, increasing the likelihood of protein fermentation in the colon. This process generates ammonia, hydrogen sulfide, biogenic amines, phenols, and indoles, which irritate the intestinal lining and impair epithelial integrity. Egg fats slow gastric emptying, compounding digestive inefficiency and increasing fermentation burden.

Microbiome & Gut Ecology

Egg consumption favors proteolytic and acid-forming bacteria over carbohydrate-fermenting species. This microbial shift reduces short-chain fatty acid production and increases toxic secondary metabolites. Dysbiosis contributes to intestinal permeability and systemic inflammation.

Immune System

Partially digested egg proteins and endotoxins crossing the gut barrier activate immune pathways. Repeated exposure promotes chronic low-grade inflammation, immune fatigue, and molecular mimicry. Egg-derived antigens may provoke immune confusion rather than resolution.

Metabolic System

Egg fats contribute to intramyocellular lipid accumulation, impairing insulin signaling. Dietary cholesterol increases oxidative stress and lipid dysregulation. Endotoxin absorption further worsens insulin resistance and metabolic inflammation.

Cardiovascular System

Egg-derived cholesterol and TMAO formation promote endothelial dysfunction, arterial plaque development, and increased coronary artery calcium scores. Chronic inflammation accelerates vascular aging.

Neurological System

Gut-derived inflammatory compounds influence neurotransmitter balance and blood–brain barrier integrity. Neuroinflammation manifests as brain fog, fatigue, mood instability, and cognitive decline.

Hormonal and Endocrine Systems

Egg consumption influences steroid hormone signaling and IGF-1 pathways, promoting growth signaling over repair. Hormonal disruption contributes to cancer risk and metabolic dysregulation.

Appendix C: Common Egg Claims vs Biological Reality

Egg-related nutrition claims persist largely through repetition. Below is a comparison between common assertions and what biology demonstrates.

• **Claim:** Eggs are the perfect protein.

• **Reality:** Protein quality scoring does not account for digestion, fermentation, endotoxin absorption, or inflammatory cost. Amino acids are abundantly available from plant foods without these burdens.

• **Claim:** Eggs are essential for choline.

• **Reality:** Choline is widely available in cruciferous vegetables, legumes, seeds, and greens. Plant-based choline does not promote TMAO formation.

• **Claim:** Eggs are safe if eaten raw.

• **Reality:** Raw eggs introduce avidin, enzyme inhibitors, increased antigenicity, and greater protein fermentation independent of bacterial contamination.

• **Claim:** Eggs are heart-healthy.

• **Reality:** Egg consumption is associated with increased coronary artery calcium, cardiovascular disease risk, and stroke incidence.

• **Claim:** Eggs are good for diabetics.

• **Reality:** Egg consumption is consistently associated with increased risk of type 2 diabetes and worsened insulin resistance.

• **Claim:** Eggs are natural and therefore healthy.

• **Reality:** Natural origin does not equal biological compatibility. Eggs are reproductive tissue, not maintenance nutrition.

Appendix D: Egg-Related Risks by Condition

This appendix summarizes populations most affected by egg consumption:

• Individuals with insulin resistance or diabetes experience worsened glycemic control, increased lipid accumulation, and higher cardiovascular risk.

• Individuals with autoimmune conditions may experience heightened immune activation, inflammatory flares, and symptom persistence.

• Individuals with digestive disorders often experience bloating, gas, dysbiosis, and intestinal permeability exacerbation.

• Individuals with cardiovascular disease or risk factors demonstrate increased atherosclerotic progression and endothelial dysfunction.

• Children may experience increased immune sensitivity, neuroinflammation, and hormonal disruption during development.

• Older adults experience compounded oxidative stress, inflammatory burden, and metabolic decline.

Appendix E: Frequently Asked Questions

Do I need eggs to get enough protein?

No. The body assembles proteins from amino acids, which are abundant in whole plant foods when caloric intake and variety are sufficient.

Will removing eggs make me weak or hungry?

Most people experience improved energy and lighter satiety once digestion and inflammation improve.

What about athletes?

Athletes often experience improved recovery and endurance when inflammation and endotoxin exposure are reduced.

Is occasional egg consumption harmful?

Occasional exposure is less problematic than daily intake. Frequency, not singular consumption, drives cumulative harm.

How long until I feel benefits after removing eggs?

Digestive and cognitive improvements are often noticed within weeks, while metabolic and inflammatory improvements accrue over months.

Epilogue: What Remains After the Egg

When a long-held belief dissolves, something quieter often takes place. This is not certainty or triumph, but space in the body, mind, and relationship between hunger and trust. This book primarily teaches us to restore the capacity to listen.

Our intention is not convincing the reader to abandon a single food. We are encouraging you to feel the difference between nourishment and burden. To recognize when the body sighs with relief rather than bracing for digestion.

Eggs, like many foods before them, asked to be re-examined. Not to be judged or demonized but seen clearly. When that seeing happens, the decision is often made. What once felt necessary begins to feel unnecessary. What once felt normal begins to feel heavy.

Health often arrives as quiet coherence. We recognize our health shifting when digestion becomes simple again, energy steadies, inflammation softens, and the body stops negotiating and starts trusting. These shifts do not announce themselves loudly. They are recognized only by those willing to notice subtlety.

Nothing in nature is wrong for existing as is. Eggs are not mistakes. They are exquisite reproductive vessels, perfectly designed for the task they were meant to fulfill. The confusion begins only when function is displaced, as when growth foods are asked to serve maintenance, when density replaces rhythm, and when habit replaces listening.

This book closes not with rules, but with an invitation to return to discernment. Our body remembers what we are built for. When the noise quiets, guidance returns. The way has always known.

A Note from the Authors

We wrote this book to complete a conservation and present clean facts that are not persuaded by monetary gains. We are not here to win an argument.

The Meat Effect, Dirty Dairy, and now *The Bad Egg* form a trilogy of clarification. Each book asked the same question in a different form: *What happens inside the human body when this food becomes routine?* Each answer emerged not from ideology, but from biology, pattern recognition, and lived experience.

We recognize that food is personal and is shaped by culture, memory, survival, and identity. Questioning a familiar food can feel unsettling and even threatening. If this book stirred resistance, that response is understandable. If the contents stirred relief, that response is equally meaningful.

Our hope is not that every reader arrives at the same conclusion, but that each reader feels empowered to investigate honestly and to listen to their own body with curiosity rather than obedience. No authority replaces lived coherence. No study outweighs sustained clarity.

Health is not found in purity, restriction, or perfection but in alignment. In choosing foods that do not require defense. In letting nourishment feel like support rather than effort. If this book helped restore even a small measure of trust between you and your body, then we have fulfilled our purpose. We respect your journey and have faith in the body's wisdom.

Author's Note

For more than fifteen years, Anthony and I have lived completely plant-based. I have also been eating all organic, and have abstained from alcohol, pills, or stimulants of any kind. This path of purity was never a doctrine for us but was more of a discovery that revealed, over time, how the human body, when aligned with nature's design, begins to hum again with clarity. Energy ceases to be borrowed from stimulants or stolen from other beings and becomes self-generating, luminous, and steady.

The words in *The Meat Effect* were born from that lived experience. They are not theories written from distance, but reflections from within the process of watching the blood brighten, the mind clear, the emotions steady, and the sense of life expand beyond the body.

I have witnessed, both personally and through the work at SoulSpire: The Healing Playground, how purification reawakens intelligence. When the body is freed from chemical noise, we begin to listen again to the pulse of Earth, to intuition, and to the quiet guidance of Spirit. Healing becomes not something we *do*, but something we *allow*.

To live grain-free, plant-based, and free of alcohol or pharmaceuticals is not asceticism but is sovereignty. We embody the joy of knowing that the body's equilibrium depends not on consumption but on coherence. This is the living proof that the body, like the planet, can be restored once interference ends.

May these pages serve as both reminder and invitation that each of us holds the same innate ability to regenerate, awaken, and live as light remembers, being clean, conscious, and free.

About the Authors

Jesse Jacoby is a dedicated father, expressionist, and advocate for compassion, equanimity, and purity. He expends energy adventuring in forests, creating, learning, playing, and writing. He has been following an all organic, fully plant-based, grain-free, oil-free, and alcohol-free lifestyle for fifteen years.

Jesse is the founder and CEO of Soulspire: The Healing Playground (*soulspire.com*). This is a biohacking and purification center with locations near Lake Tahoe in Truckee, CA, and in Nevada City, CA.

Jesse is the author of The Raw Cure: Healing Beyond Medicine (1st & 2nd Editions), The Way Knows, The Meat Effect, Dirty Dairy, You Are Not Powerless, Sovereign Biology, The Frequency Diet, Eating Plant-Based, and several other nonfiction titles. He and his children have also co-authored several kids' books implementing values and raising awareness around compassion and mindfulness.

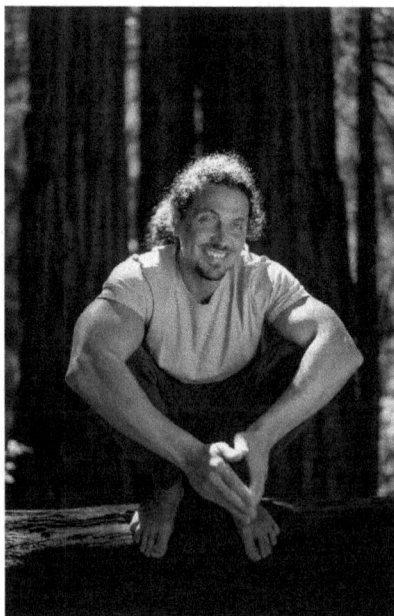

About the Authors

Born in Newcastle, UK, and now 45 years into a life defined by curiosity and evolution, Anthony Lowther has spent nearly three decades exploring the frontiers of human health. His journey from committed carnivore to devoted vegan, and from experimenter to embodiment reflects a rare level of rigor, humility, and lived inquiry.

Since the age of sixteen, Anthony has treated his body as a living laboratory, testing hypotheses, tracking outcomes, and observing how food becomes chemistry, chemistry becomes energy, and energy becomes the quality of a human life. For thirty years he explored the effects of a meat-heavy diet with scientific precision, then fifteen years ago pivoted into veganism with the same disciplined curiosity. His transition was a conscious choice rooted in ethics, physiology, and a deepening sense of responsibility to all living beings.

Anthony's work sits at the intersection of science, compassion, and systemic thinking. He is a practitioner who translates research into practical daily habits, a scientist who measures outcomes rather than opinions, and an advocate for a world in which human health and planetary health are no longer at odds. His guiding philosophy is simple yet profound, teaching that what sustains us must nourish all life, including humans, animals, and the ecosystems that hold us.

As a global community leader, Anthony has facilitated hundreds of retreats around the world, cultivating transformation for groups ranging from intimate circles of fifteen to celebratory gatherings of three hundred. He is also the founder of RISE & SHINE, a sober celebration platform where clarity, presence, and joy replace the distractions of modern culture.

Anthony's ambition is as bold as sincere. He aims to help create a system that works for all life while continually becoming the healthiest, most compassionate version of himself. His evolution is ongoing, measured weekly, lived fully, and shared openly. His life's work is a testament to continuous refinement, expanding consciousness, and an unwavering commitment to peace, vitality, and systemic harmony.

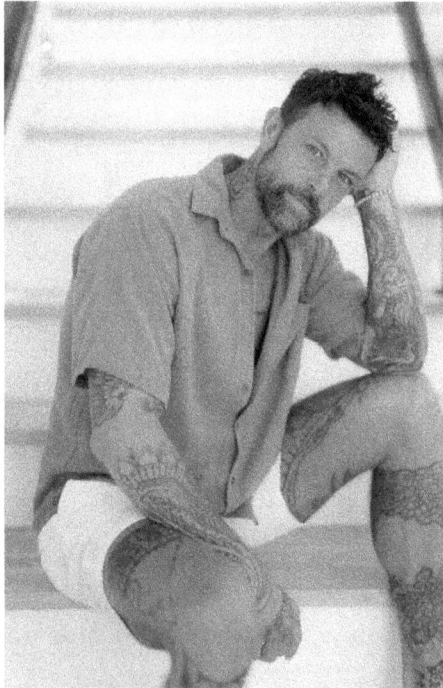

Bibliography

Lesson 1:

• Appleby, Paul N., et al. "Dietary Patterns and Cardiovascular Disease Risk." *The American Journal of Clinical Nutrition*, vol. 95, no. 2, 2012, pp. 395–403.

• Barnard, Neal D., et al. "Dietary Cholesterol and Cardiovascular Risk: A Review." *Nutrition Reviews*, vol. 77, no. 8, 2019, pp. 537–549.

• Carroll, Aaron E. "The Trouble with Nutrition Science." *The New York Times*, 1 May 2019.

• Nestle, Marion. *Food Politics: How the Food Industry Influences Nutrition and Health*. University of California Press, 2013.

• U.S. Department of Agriculture. *Egg Products and Food Labeling Practices*. USDA Economic Research Service, 2018.

• Williams, Peter G. "Breakfast and the Diet." *Nutrition & Dietetics*, vol. 71, no. 1, 2014, pp. 1–3.

Lesson 2:

• Campbell, T. Colin, and Thomas M. Campbell II. *The China Study*. BenBella Books, 2005.

• Cordain, Loren. *The Paleo Diet*. John Wiley & Sons, 2002.

• Milner, John A. "Dietary Proteins and Cellular Proliferation." *The Journal of Nutrition*, vol. 134, no. 6, 2004, pp. 1486S–1490S.

• Popkin, Barry M. "The Nutrition Transition and Its Health Implications." *Public Health Nutrition*, vol. 8, no. 6A, 2005, pp. 724–732.

• Trowell, Hugh. "Refined Carbohydrates and Disease." *Academic Press*, 1975.

Lesson 3:

• Fontana, Luigi, et al. "Protein Intake, IGF-1, and Longevity." *Cell Metabolism,* vol. 14, no. 3, 2011, pp. 349–352.

• Mariotti, François. "Plant Protein, Animal Protein, and Protein Quality." *The Journal of Nutrition,* vol. 147, no. 7, 2017, pp. 1441S–1447S.

• Millward, D. Joe. "An Adaptive Metabolic Demand Model for Protein." *The American Journal of Clinical Nutrition,* vol. 87, no. 5, 2008, pp. 1554S–1561S.

• Tomé, Daniel, and Claire Bos. "Amino Acid Bioavailability and Utilization." *The American Journal of Clinical Nutrition,* vol. 91, no. 3, 2010, pp. 709S–713S.

• Windey, Karen, et al. "Protein Fermentation and Gut Health." *Current Opinion in Clinical Nutrition and Metabolic Care,* vol. 15, no. 1, 2012, pp. 79–86.

Lesson 4:

• Boye, Joyce I., et al. "Factors Affecting Protein Digestibility." *Food Research International,* vol. 44, no. 10, 2011, pp. 3234–3241.

• Kato, A., and K. Takahashi. "Egg Protein Digestibility and Structure." *Journal of Agricultural and Food Chemistry,* vol. 44, no. 1, 1996, pp. 17–22.

• Windey, Karen, et al. "Protein Fermentation and Gut Health." *Current Opinion in Clinical Nutrition and Metabolic Care,* vol. 15, no. 1, 2012, pp. 79–86.

Lesson 5:

• Said, Hamid M. "Biotin Bioavailability and Intestinal Absorption." *The American Journal of Clinical Nutrition,* vol. 63, no. 4, 1996, pp. 491–498.

• Whitney, Eleanor, and Sharon Rolfes. *Understanding Nutrition.* Cengage Learning, 2018.

• Kopper, Robert A., et al. "Food Protein-Induced Enterocolitis." *The Journal of Allergy and Clinical Immunology*, vol. 129, no. 1, 2012, pp. 36–44.

Lesson 6:
• Smith, E. A., and G. T. Macfarlane. "Protein Fermentation in the Colon." *Anaerobe*, vol. 3, no. 5, 1997, pp. 327–337.
• Roediger, W. E. "Role of Anaerobic Bacteria in Colonic Health." *Gut*, vol. 21, no. 9, 1980, pp. 793–798.
• Remer, Thomas, and Friedrich Manz. "Potential Renal Acid Load of Foods." *The American Journal of Clinical Nutrition*, vol. 73, no. 6, 2001, pp. 1181–1182.

Lesson 7:
• Windey, Karen, et al. "Protein Fermentation and Gut-Derived Metabolites." *Current Opinion in Clinical Nutrition and Metabolic Care*, vol. 15, no. 1, 2012, pp. 79–86.
• Davila, Anne-Marie, et al. "Intestinal Luminal Metabolites." *Gut Microbes*, vol. 4, no. 2, 2013, pp. 95–109.
• Knecht, Heike, et al. "Gut-Derived Phenolic Compounds." *Journal of Nutrition*, vol. 134, no. 6, 2004, pp. 1526–1532.

Lesson 8:
• Cani, Patrice D., et al. "Metabolic Endotoxemia and Insulin Resistance." *Diabetes*, vol. 56, no. 7, 2007, pp. 1761–1772.
• Fukui, Hiroshi. "Increased Intestinal Permeability." *World Journal of Gastroenterology*, vol. 22, no. 17, 2016, pp. 4681–4687.
• Ghoshal, S., et al. "Dietary Fat and Endotoxin Absorption." *Journal of Lipid Research*, vol. 50, no. 1, 2009, pp. 90–97.

Lesson 9:

• Hunt, James N., and M. T. Stubbs. "The Control of Gastric Emptying." *The Journal of Physiology*, vol. 245, no. 1, 1975, pp. 209–225.

• Ghoshal, S., et al. "Chylomicrons and Endotoxin Absorption." *Journal of Lipid Research*, vol. 50, no. 1, 2009, pp. 90–97.

• Feinle-Bisset, Christine, and N. W. Read. "Fat-Induced Slowing of Gastric Emptying." *The American Journal of Clinical Nutrition*, vol. 77, no. 1, 2003, pp. 4–10.

Lesson 10:

• Staprans, Ilia, et al. "Oxidized Cholesterol in the Diet." *The American Journal of Clinical Nutrition*, vol. 69, no. 1, 1999, pp. 13–22.

• Brown, Michael S., and Joseph L. Goldstein. "A Receptor-Mediated Pathway for Cholesterol Homeostasis." *Science*, vol. 232, no. 4746, 1986, pp. 34–47.

• Wang, Zeneng, et al. "Gut Flora Metabolism of Phosphatidylcholine." *Nature*, vol. 472, no. 7341, 2011, pp. 57–63.

Lesson 11:

• Shulman, Gerald I. "Cellular Mechanisms of Insulin Resistance." *The Journal of Clinical Investigation*, vol. 106, no. 2, 2000, pp. 171–176.

• Pan, An, et al. "Egg Consumption and Risk of Type 2 Diabetes." *The American Journal of Clinical Nutrition*, vol. 98, no. 1, 2013, pp. 146–152.

• Samuel, Varman T., and Gerald I. Shulman. "The Pathogenesis of Insulin Resistance." *Cell*, vol. 148, no. 5, 2012, pp. 852–871.

Lesson 12:

• Friedman, Mendel. "Protein Structure and Heat-Induced Chemical Changes." *Journal of Agricultural and Food Chemistry*, vol. 42, no. 1, 1994, pp. 2–8.
• Mills, E. N. C., et al. "Impact of Food Processing on Protein Allergenicity." *Molecular Nutrition & Food Research*, vol. 53, no. 8, 2009, pp. 963–969.
• Wedzicha, Barbara L., and David S. Mottram. "Heat-Induced Changes in Food Proteins." *Food Chemistry*, vol. 75, no. 3, 2001, pp. 299–305.

Lesson 13:

• Uribarri, Jaime, et al. "Advanced Glycation End Products in Foods." *Journal of the American Dietetic Association*, vol. 110, no. 6, 2010, pp. 911–916.
• Goldberg, T., et al. "Advanced Glycoxidation End Products." *The Journal of Clinical Endocrinology & Metabolism*, vol. 89, no. 2, 2004, pp. 709–716.
• Vlassara, Helen, and Gary E. Striker. "AGEs and Inflammation." *Annals of the New York Academy of Sciences*, vol. 1126, 2008, pp. 106–112.

Lesson 14:

• Varki, Ajit. "Human Sialic Acid Biology and Pathology." *Proceedings of the National Academy of Sciences*, vol. 108, no. 28, 2011, pp. 11329–11336.
• Samraj, Ankur N., et al. "Dietary Neu5Gc and Human Inflammation." *Proceedings of the National Academy of Sciences*, vol. 112, no. 2, 2015, pp. 542–547.
• Padler-Karavani, Vered, et al. "Neu5Gc and Cancer Risk." *Glycobiology*, vol. 21, no. 1, 2011, pp. 44–56.

Lesson 15:

• Djoussé, Luc, and J. Michael Gaziano. "Egg Consumption and Risk of Heart Failure." *Circulation,* vol. 122, no. 5, 2010, pp. 506–511.

• Shin, Jae Eun, et al. "Egg Consumption and Coronary Artery Calcium." *Atherosclerosis,* vol. 267, 2017, pp. 63–69.

• Wang, Zeneng, et al. "Trimethylamine-N-Oxide and Cardiovascular Risk." *The New England Journal of Medicine,* vol. 368, no. 17, 2013, pp. 1575–1584.

Lesson 16:

• Pan, An, et al. "Egg Consumption and Risk of Type 2 Diabetes." *The American Journal of Clinical Nutrition,* vol. 98, no. 1, 2013, pp. 146–152.

• Djoussé, Luc, et al. "Egg Consumption and Diabetes Risk." *The American Journal of Clinical Nutrition,* vol. 93, no. 2, 2011, pp. 390–397.

• Uribarri, Jaime, et al. "Advanced Glycation End Products and Diabetes." *Current Diabetes Reports,* vol. 15, no. 12, 2015, p. 123.

Lesson 17:

• Missmer, Stacey A., et al. "Meat and Egg Consumption and Breast Cancer Risk." *International Journal of Cancer,* vol. 109, no. 4, 2004, pp. 593–600.

• Richman, Erin L., et al. "Egg Consumption and Prostate Cancer Progression." *Cancer Prevention Research,* vol. 4, no. 12, 2011, pp. 2110–2117.

• Fontana, Luigi, et al. "Dietary Protein and Cancer Risk." *Cell Metabolism,* vol. 14, no. 3, 2011, pp. 349–352.

Lesson 18:

• Zhong, Victor W., et al. "Associations of Dietary Cholesterol and Egg Consumption with Mortality." *JAMA,* vol. 321, no. 11, 2019, pp. 1081–1095.

• Orlich, Michael J., et al. "Vegetarian Dietary Patterns and Mortality." *JAMA Internal Medicine,* vol. 173, no. 13, 2013, pp. 1230–1238.

• Barnard, Neal D. "Dietary Cholesterol and Longevity." *Nutrition Reviews,* vol. 75, no. 3, 2017, pp. 173–185.

Lesson 19:

• Grohskopf, Lisa A., et al. "Prevention and Control of Seasonal Influenza." *MMWR Recommendations and Reports,* vol. 69, no. 8, 2020, pp. 1–24.

• Nachbagauer, Rino, and Florian Krammer. "Influenza Virus Cultivation in Eggs." *Viruses,* vol. 9, no. 9, 2017, p. 276.

• Dimitrov, Dimiter S. "Therapeutic Proteins." *Methods in Molecular Biology,* vol. 899, 2012, pp. 1–26.

Lesson 20:

• Cusick, Matthew F., et al. "Molecular Mimicry in Autoimmune Disease." *Clinical Reviews in Allergy & Immunology,* vol. 42, no. 1, 2012, pp. 102–111.

• Fasano, Alessio. "Leaky Gut and Autoimmune Disease." *Clinical Reviews in Allergy & Immunology,* vol. 42, no. 1, 2012, pp. 71–78.

• Vojdani, Aristo. "Reaction of the Immune System to Dietary Proteins." *Journal of Applied Microbiology,* vol. 102, no. 4, 2007, pp. 1109–1118.

Lesson 21:

• Hotamisligil, Gökhan S. "Inflammation and Metabolic Disorders." *Nature,* vol. 444, no. 7121, 2006, pp. 860–867.

• Libby, Peter. "Inflammation in Atherosclerosis." *Nature,* vol. 420, no. 6917, 2002, pp. 868–874.

• Calder, Philip C. "Dietary Factors and Chronic Inflammation." *Proceedings of the Nutrition Society,* vol. 72, no. 3, 2013, pp. 326–335.

Lesson 22:

• Vojdani, Aristo, and Elroy Vojdani. "Food Sensitivities and Immune Reactivity." *Alternative Therapies in Health and Medicine,* vol. 21, no. 2, 2015, pp. 18–31.

• Petersen, Christine, et al. "Dietary Proteins and Gut Immune Activation." *Nutrients,* vol. 9, no. 6, 2017, p. 584.

• Cryan, John F., and Timothy G. Dinan. "Mind-Altering Microorganisms." *Nature Reviews Neuroscience,* vol. 13, no. 10, 2012, pp. 701–712.

Lesson 23:

• McEwen, Bruce S. "Protective and Damaging Effects of Stress Mediators." *The New England Journal of Medicine,* vol. 338, no. 3, 1998, pp. 171–179.

• Hotamisligil, Gökhan S. "Inflammation and Metabolic Disorders." *Nature,* vol. 444, no. 7121, 2006, pp. 860–867.

• Kotas, Mark E., and Ruslan Medzhitov. "Homeostasis, Inflammation, and Disease." *Cell,* vol. 160, no. 5, 2015, pp. 816–827.

Lesson 24:

• Prescott, Susan L. "Early-Life Environmental Determinants of Allergic Diseases." *Clinical & Experimental Allergy,* vol. 40, no. 8, 2010, pp. 1217–1229.

• Borre, Yoanna E., et al. "Microbiota and Neurodevelopment." *Trends in Neurosciences,* vol. 37, no. 7, 2014, pp. 407–417.

• Gleeson, Michael, et al. "Nutrition and Immune Function in Children." *British Journal of Nutrition,* vol. 96, no. S3, 2006, pp. S75–S81.

Lesson 25:

• Campbell, T. Colin, and Thomas M. Campbell II. *The China Study.* BenBella Books, 2005.

• Orlich, Michael J., et al. "Vegetarian Dietary Patterns and Mortality." *JAMA Internal Medicine*, vol. 173, no. 13, 2013, pp. 1230–1238.

• Thorning, T. K., et al. "Whole Dairy Matrix and Health." *The American Journal of Clinical Nutrition*, vol. 105, no. 5, 2017, pp. 1033–1045.

Lesson 26:

• Nestle, Marion. *Food Politics*. University of California Press, 2013.

• Zhong, Victor W., et al. "Dietary Cholesterol and Mortality." *JAMA*, vol. 321, no. 11, 2019, pp. 1081–1095.

• Popkin, Barry M. "Nutrition Transition." *Public Health Nutrition*, vol. 8, no. 6A, 2005, pp. 724–732.

Lesson 27:

• Ludwig, David S., et al. "Dietary Patterns and Long-Term Health." *The BMJ*, vol. 356, 2017, j416.

• McEwen, Bruce S. "Allostatic Load." *Annals of the New York Academy of Sciences*, vol. 840, 1998, pp. 33–44.

• Hu, Frank B. "Dietary Patterns and Chronic Disease." *The New England Journal of Medicine*, vol. 350, no. 10, 2004, pp. 1084–1096.

Lesson 28:

• Mariotti, François. "Plant Protein, Animal Protein, and Protein Quality." *The Journal of Nutrition*, vol. 147, no. 7, 2017, pp. 1441S–1447S.

• Millward, D. Joe. "An Adaptive Metabolic Demand Model for Protein." *The American Journal of Clinical Nutrition*, vol. 87, no. 5, 2008, pp. 1554S–1561S.

• Campbell, T. Colin. *Whole: Rethinking the Science of Nutrition*. BenBella Books, 2013.

Lesson 29:

• Zeisel, Steven H., and Kerry-Ann da Costa. "Choline: An Essential Nutrient." *The American Journal of Clinical Nutrition*, vol. 79, no. 1, 2004, pp. 7–12.

• Said, Hamid M. "Biotin Bioavailability." *The American Journal of Clinical Nutrition*, vol. 63, no. 4, 1996, pp. 491–498.

• Craig, Winston J. "Health Effects of Vegan Diets." *The American Journal of Clinical Nutrition*, vol. 89, no. 5, 2009, pp. 1627S–1633S.

Lesson 30:

• Ludwig, David S. "The Glycemic Index." *JAMA*, vol. 287, no. 18, 2002, pp. 2414–2423.

• Barnard, Neal D., et al. "Plant-Based Diets and Energy Metabolism." *Nutrition Reviews*, vol. 77, no. 4, 2019, pp. 259–268.

• Esselstyn, Caldwell B. *Prevent and Reverse Heart Disease*. Avery, 2007.

Lesson 31:

• Milner, John A. "Dietary Signals and Cellular Growth." *The Journal of Nutrition*, vol. 134, no. 6, 2004, pp. 1486S–1490S.

• Cordain, Loren. *The Paleo Diet*. Wiley, 2002.

• Lieberman, Daniel E. *The Story of the Human Body*. Pantheon Books, 2013.

Lesson32:

• Illich, Ivan. *Medical Nemesis*. Pantheon Books, 1976.

• Nestle, Marion. *Food Politics*. University of California Press, 2013.

• Kabat-Zinn, Jon. *Full Catastrophe Living*. Bantam, 1990.

Lesson 33:

• Berry, Wendell. *The Unsettling of America*. Sierra Club Books, 1977.

- Kimmerer, Robin Wall. *Braiding Sweetgrass*. Milkweed Editions, 2013.
- Trungpa, Chögyam. *Cutting Through Spiritual Materialism*. Shambhala, 1973.

Lesson 34:
- Zhong, Victor W., et al. "Associations of Dietary Cholesterol and Egg Consumption with Mortality." *JAMA*, vol. 321, no. 11, 2019, pp. 1081–1095.
- Pan, An, et al. "Egg Consumption and Risk of Type 2 Diabetes." *The American Journal of Clinical Nutrition*, vol. 98, no. 1, 2013, pp. 146–152.
- Uribarri, Jaime, et al. "Advanced Glycation End Products in Foods." *Journal of the American Dietetic Association*, vol. 110, no. 6, 2010, pp. 911–916.

Lesson 35:
- Hotamisligil, Gökhan S. "Inflammation and Metabolic Disorders." *Nature*, vol. 444, no. 7121, 2006, pp. 860–867.
- Prescott, Susan L. "Early-Life Determinants of Immune Health." *Clinical & Experimental Allergy*, vol. 40, no. 8, 2010, pp. 1217–1229.
- Fasano, Alessio. "Leaky Gut and Autoimmune Disease." *Clinical Reviews in Allergy & Immunology*, vol. 42, no. 1, 2012, pp. 71–78.

Lesson 36:
- Illich, Ivan. *Medical Nemesis*. Pantheon Books, 1976.
- Kabat-Zinn, Jon. *Wherever You Go, There You Are*. Hyperion, 1994.
- Berry, Wendell. *The Unsettling of America*. Sierra Club Books, 1977.

Substance Shield
Ally of the Aftermath

Substance Shield is a botanical supplement line born from the wisdom of The High Life, a guide for conscious living in a chemically saturated world. Our products exist to support the body's resilience before and after exposure to substances, offering tools of renewal, not judgment. Whether facing pharmaceutical fallout, recreational recovery, or environmental residue, our mission is to replenish what modern life strips away.

Every formula is organic, vegan, wild-harvested, and crafted from whole foods, roots, and ancient botanicals designed to support detoxification pathways, restore depleted micronutrients, and aid in cellular resilience.

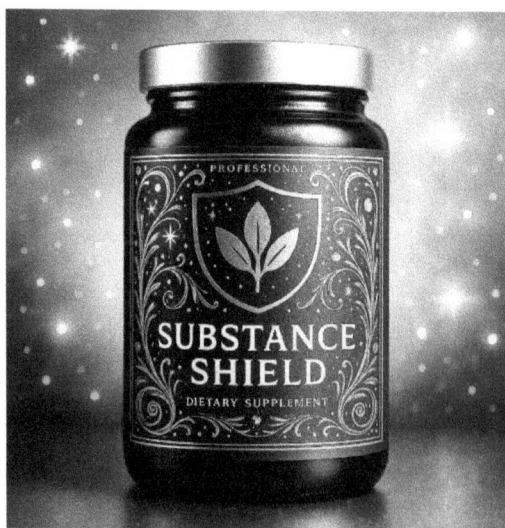

www.substanceshield.com
Instagram: @substanceshield

SOUL◉SPIRE
The Healing Playground

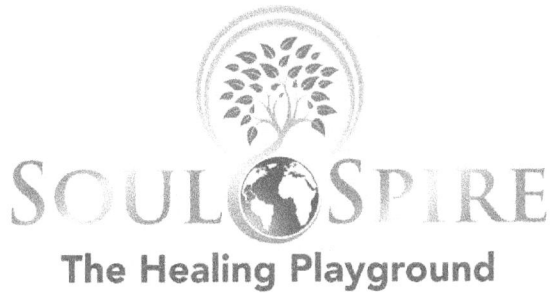

Soulspire is a biohacking and purification offering with centers located in Truckee, CA, and Nevada City, CA which provides each of the biohacking tools suggested in this guide for regenerating the body before and after substance use.

Access the site www.soulspire.com

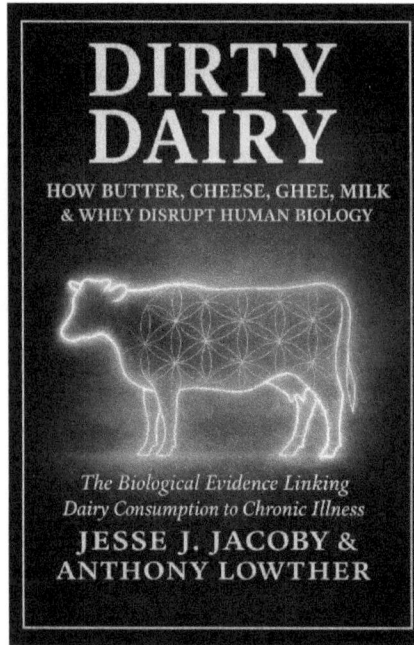

DIRTY DAIRY

HOW BUTTER, CHEESE, GHEE, MILK
& WHEY DISRUPT HUMAN BIOLOGY

*The Biological Evidence Linking
Dairy Consumption to Chronic Illness*

JESSE J. JACOBY &
ANTHONY LOWTHER

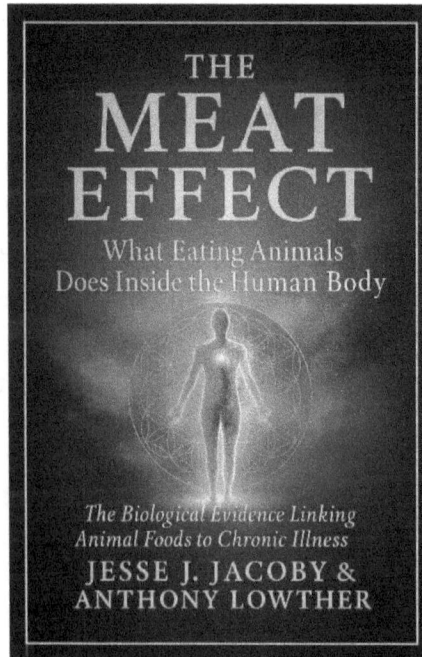

THE

MEAT
EFFECT

What Eating Animals
Does Inside the Human Body

*The Biological Evidence Linking
Animal Foods to Chronic Illness*

JESSE J. JACOBY &
ANTHONY LOWTHER

www.ingramcontent.com/pod-product-compliance
Lightning Source LLC
Chambersburg PA
CBHW081409270326
41931CB00016B/3430